Tasty Dishe
Vegan Diet

A Cooking Guide to Improve your Vegan Recipes

Meadow Lambert

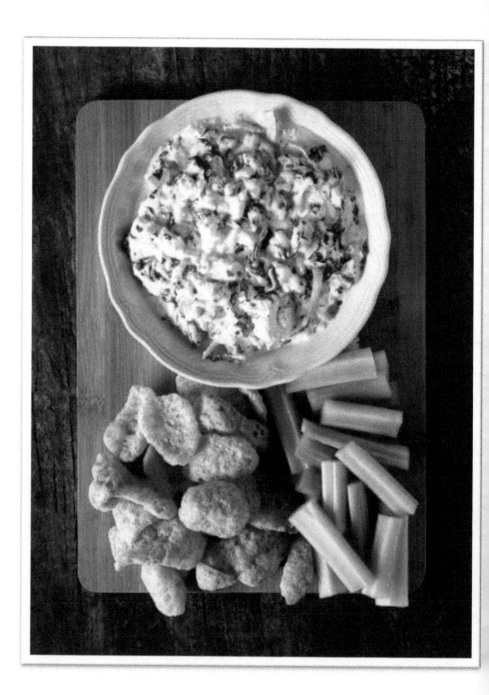

by reading this document, the reader agrees that under no circumstances is the author responsible for any losses, direct or indirect, which are incurred as a result of the use of information contained within this document, including, but not limited to, — errors, omissions, or inaccuracies.

Table of Contents

Mint Chocolate Protein Smoothie

Preparation Time: 5 minutes

Cooking Time: 0 minutes

Servings: 4

Ingredients:

- 4 tablespoons ground flaxseed

- 4 cups fresh spinach

- 4 frozen banana, sliced

- 4 scoops of chocolate protein powder

- 4 tablespoons chopped dark chocolate, vegan

- ½ cup melted dark chocolate

- 1 teaspoon peppermint extract, unsweetened

- 4 tablespoons honey

- 3 cups almond milk, unsweetened

- 1 cup ice cubed

Directions:

1. Add all the ingredients in the order into a food processor or blender and then pulse for 1 to 2 minutes until blended, scraping the sides of the container frequently.

2. Distribute the smoothie among glasses and then serve.

Nutrition: 480.5 Cal 20.3 g Fat 8.4 g Saturated Fat 45.6 g Carbohydrates 9.7 g Fiber 22.5 g Sugars 31.2 g Protein

Sunrise Smoothie

Preparation Time: 5 minutes

Cooking Time: 0 minutes

Servings: 4

Ingredients:

- 4 tablespoons chia seed

- 2 frozen banana

- 2 lemon, peeled

- 2 cups diced carrots

- 4 clementine, peeled

- 4 cups frozen strawberries, unsweetened

- 12 tablespoons pomegranate tendrils

- 2 cup almond milk, unsweetened

Directions:

1. Add all the ingredients in the order into a food processor or blender and then pulse for 1 to 2 minutes until blended, scraping the sides of the container frequently.

2. Distribute the smoothie among glasses and then serve.

Nutrition: 274 Cal 5.4 g Fat 0.5 g Saturated Fat 57.3 g Carbohydrates 13.3 g Fiber 33.8 g Sugars 0.5 g Protein

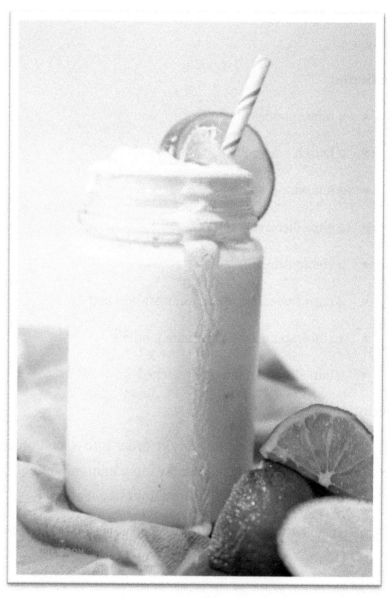

Sunshine Orange Smoothie

reparation Time: 5 minutes

ooking Time: 0 minutes

ervings: 4

1gredients:

- 2 medium oranges, zested, juiced
- 4 frozen bananas
- 4 tablespoons goji berries
- ½ cup hemp seeds
- 1 teaspoon grated ginger
- 1 cup almond milk, unsweetened
- ½ cup of ice cubes

)irections:

1. Add all the ingredients in the order into a food processor or blender and then pulse for 1 to 2 minutes until blended, scraping the sides of the container frequently.

2. Distribute the smoothie among glasses and then serve.

Nutrition: 131 Cal 2.3 g Fat 0.3 g Saturated Fat 26.7 g Carbohydrates 4 g Fiber 11 g Sugars 2.6 g Protein

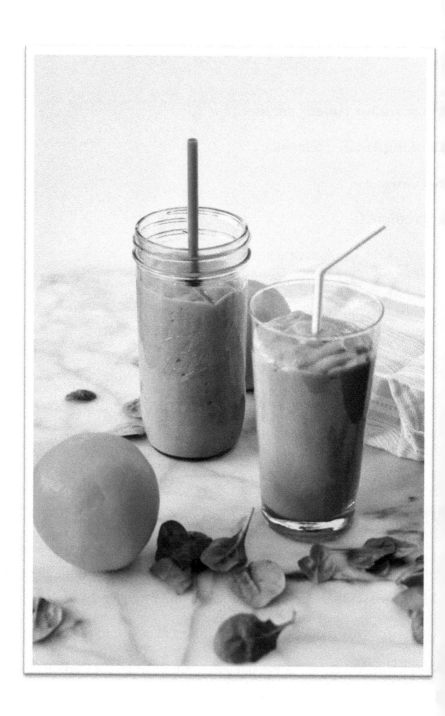

Sabich Sandwich

Preparation Time: 10 minutes

Cooking Time: 10 minutes

Servings: 4

Ingredients:

- 1/2 cup cooked white beans

- 2 medium potatoes, peeled, boiled, ½-inch thick sliced

- 1 medium eggplant, destemmed, ½-inch cubed

- 4 dill pickles, ¼-inch thick sliced

- ¼ teaspoon of sea salt

- 2 tablespoons olive oil

- 1/4 teaspoon harissa paste

- 1/2 cup hummus

- 1 tablespoon mayonnaise

- 4 pita bread pockets

- 1/2 cup tabbouleh salad

Directions:

1. Take a small frying pan, place it over medium-low heat, add oil and wait until it gets hot.

2. Season eggplant pieces with salt, add to the hot frying pan and cook for 8 minutes until softened, and when done, remove the pan from heat.

3. Take a small bowl, place white beans in it, add harissa paste and mayonnaise and then stir until combined.

4. Assemble the sandwich and for this, place pita bread on clean working space, smear generously with hummus, then cover half of each pita bread with potato slices and top with a dill pickle slices.

5. Spoon 2 tablespoons of white bean mixture on each dill pickle, top with 3 tablespoons of cooked eggplant pieces and 2 tablespoons of tabbouleh salad and then cover the filling with the other half of pita bread.

6. Serve straight away.

Nutrition: 386 Cal 13 g Fat 2 g Saturated Fat 56 g Carbohydrates 7 g Fiber 3 g Sugars 12 g Protein

Pinto Bean Stew with Cauliflower

Preparation Time: 10 min

Cooking Time: 25 min

Servings: 2

Ingredients:

- 1 cup water
- 1 teaspoon salt
- ¼ cup pinto beans
- 2 tablespoons coconut oil
- ½ small onion chopped
- 1 small zucchini chopped
- ½ teaspoon garlic powder
- 1 bay leaf
- 1 1/2 cups low sodium vegetable stock
- ½ cup steamed cauliflower
- ¼ cup grated mozzarella
- 1 tablespoon chopped fresh cilantro

Directions:

1. In a large bowl, dissolve 1 tablespoon of salt in the water. Add the pinto beans and soak at room temperature for 8 to 24 hours. Drain and rinse.

2. Select Sauté and adjust to Normal or Medium heat. Add the coconut oil to the Instant Pot and heat until shimmering. Add the onion and zucchini, and sprinkle with salt. Cook, stirring often, until the onion pieces separate and soften. Add the garlic powder and cook for about 1 minute, or until fragrant. Add the drained pinto beans, remaining ¼ teaspoon of salt, bay leaf, and vegetable stock.

3. Lock the lid into place. Select Pressure Cook or Manual, and adjust the pressure to High and the time to 15 minutes. After cooking, let the pressure release naturally for 10 minutes, then quick release any remaining pressure.

4. Unlock the lid. Stir in the cauliflower and bring to a simmer to heat it through and thicken the sauce slightly. Taste the beans and adjust the seasoning. Ladle into bowls and sprinkle with the mozzarella cheese and cilantro.

Nutrition: Calories 245, Total Fat 16. 2g, Saturated Fat 13. 7g, Cholesterol 2mg, Sodium 1745mg, Total Carbohydrate 22. 4g , Dietary Fiber 5.6g , Total Sugars 4. 5g, Protein 7.7g

Tempeh White Bean Gravy

Preparation Time: 05 min

Cooking Time: 20 min

Servings: 2

Ingredients:

- ½ cup cups vegetable broth

- ¼ cup soy sauce

- ¼ cup coconut oil

- 1 teaspoon garlic powder

- ½ cup chopped onion

- 1 cup chopped tempeh

- 1/8 teaspoon dried basil

- 1/8 teaspoon dried parsley

- 1/8 teaspoon ground black pepper

- 1 cup white beans, drained and rinsed

- Enough water

Directions:

1. Add vegetable broth, soy sauce, coconut oil, garlic powder, onion, tempeh, basil, parsley, black pepper and white beans to the Instant Pot. Pour the remaining ¼ cup water over everything.

2. Choose the soup function for 20 minutes.

3. Once done, remove the lid.

4. Serve and enjoy.

Nutrition: Calories 376, Total Fat 29. 4g, Saturated Fat 23. 6g, Cholesterol 0mg, Sodium 2233mg, Total Carbohydrate 22. 4g, Dietary Fiber 4. 9g, Total Sugars 4. 2g, Protein 9. 2g

Broccoli and Black Bean Chili

Preparation Time: 15 min

Cooking Time: 15 min

Servings: 2

Ingredients:

- ½ tablespoon coconut oil

- 1 cup broccoli

- 1 cup chopped red onions

- ½ tablespoon paprika

- 1/2 teaspoon salt

- ¼ cup tomatoes

- 1 cup black beans drained, rinsed

- ¼ chopped green chills

- ½ cup water

Directions:

1. In the Instant Pot, select Sauté; adjust to normal. Heat coconut oil in Instant Pot. Add broccoli, onions, paprika and salt; cook 8 to 10 minutes, stirring occasionally, until thoroughly cooked. Select Cancel.

2. Stir in tomatoes, black beans, chills and water. Secure lid, set pressure valve to Sealing. Select manual, cook on High pressure 5 minutes. Select Cancel. Keep pressure valve in sealing position to release pressure naturally.

Nutrition: Calories 408, Total Fat 5. 3g, Saturated Fat 3. 4g, Cholesterol 0mg, Sodium 607mg, Total Carbohydrate 70. 7g, Dietary Fiber 18. 1g, Total Sugars 6g, Protein 23. 3g

Mushroom & Broccoli Soup

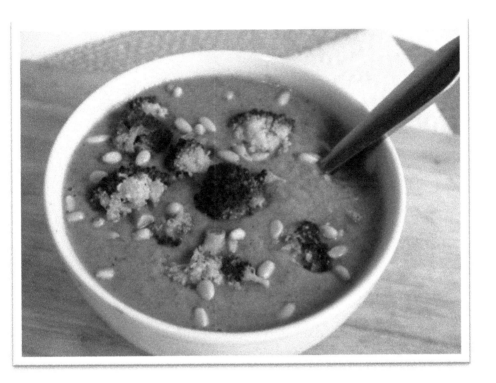

Preparation Time: 20 minutes

Cooking Time: 45 minutes

Servings: 8

Ingredients:

- 1 bundle broccoli (around 1-1/2 pounds)

- 1 tablespoon canola oil

- 1/2 pound cut crisp mushrooms

- 1 tablespoon diminished sodium soy sauce

- 2 medium carrots, finely slashed

- 2 celery ribs, finely slashed

- 1/4 cup finely slashed onion

- 1 garlic clove, minced

- 1 container (32 ounces) vegetable juices

- 2 cups of water

- 2 tablespoons lemon juice

Directions:

1. Cut broccoli florets into reduced down pieces. Strip and hack stalks.

2. In an enormous pot, heat oil over medium-high warmth; saute mushrooms until delicate, 4-6 minutes. Mix in soy sauce; expel from skillet.

3. In the same container, join broccoli stalks, carrots, celery, onion, garlic, soup, and water; heat to the point of boiling. Diminish heat; stew, revealed, until vegetables are relaxed, 25-30 minutes.

4. Puree soup utilizing a drenching blender. Or then again, cool marginally and puree the soup in a blender; come back to the dish.

5. Mix in florets and mushrooms; heat to the point of boiling. Lessen warmth to medium; cook until broccoli is delicate, 8-10 minutes, blending infrequently. Mix in lemon juice.

Nutrition: Kcal: 830 Carbohydrates: 8 g Protein: 45 g Fat: 64 g

Creamy Cauliflower Pakora Soup

Preparation Time: 20 minutes

Cooking Time: 20 minutes

Servings: 8

Ingredients:

- 1 huge head cauliflower, cut into little florets
- 5 medium potatoes, stripped and diced
- 1 huge onion, diced
- 4 medium carrots, stripped and diced
- 2 celery ribs, diced
- 1 container (32 ounces) vegetable stock
- 1 teaspoon garam masala
- 1 teaspoon garlic powder
- 1 teaspoon ground coriander
- 1 teaspoon ground turmeric
- 1 teaspoon ground cumin
- 1 teaspoon pepper

- 1 teaspoon salt

- 1/2 teaspoon squashed red pepper chips

- Water or extra vegetable stock

- New cilantro leaves

- Lime wedges, discretionary

Directions:

1. In a Dutch stove over medium-high warmth, heat initial 14 fixings to the point of boiling. Cook and mix until vegetables are delicate, around 20 minutes. Expel from heat; cool marginally. Procedure in groups in a blender or nourishment processor until smooth. Modify consistency as wanted with water (or extra stock). Sprinkle with new cilantro. Serve hot, with lime wedges whenever wanted.

2. Stop alternative: Before including cilantro, solidify cooled soup in cooler compartments. To utilize, in part defrost in cooler medium-term.

3. Warmth through in a pan, blending every so often and including a little water if fundamental. Sprinkle with cilantro. Whenever wanted, present with lime wedges.

Nutrition: Kcal: 248 Carbohydrates: 7 g Protein: 1 g Fat: 19 g

Garden Vegetable and Herb Soup

Preparation Time: 20 minutes

Cooking Time: 30 minutes

Servings: 8

Ingredients:

- 2 tablespoons olive oil

- 2 medium onions, hacked

- 2 huge carrots, cut

- 1 pound red potatoes (around 3 medium), cubed

- 2 cups of water

- 1 can (14-1/2 ounces) diced tomatoes in sauce

- 1-1/2 cups vegetable soup

- 1-1/2 teaspoons garlic powder

- 1 teaspoon dried basil

- 1/2 teaspoon salt

- 1/2 teaspoon paprika

- 1/4 teaspoon dill weed

- 1/4 teaspoon pepper

- 1 medium yellow summer squash, split and cut

- 1 medium zucchini, split and cut

Directions:

1. In a huge pan, heat oil over medium warmth. Include onions and carrots; cook and mix until onions are delicate, 4-6 minutes. Include potatoes and cook 2 minutes. Mix in water, tomatoes, juices, and seasonings.

2. Heat to the point of boiling. Diminish heat; stew, revealed, until potatoes and carrots are delicate, 9 minutes.

3. Include yellow squash and zucchini; cook until vegetables are delicate, 9 minutes longer. Serve or, whenever wanted, puree blend in clusters, including extra stock until desired consistency is accomplished.

Nutrition: Kcal: 252 Carbohydrates: 12 g Protein: 1 g Fat: 11 g

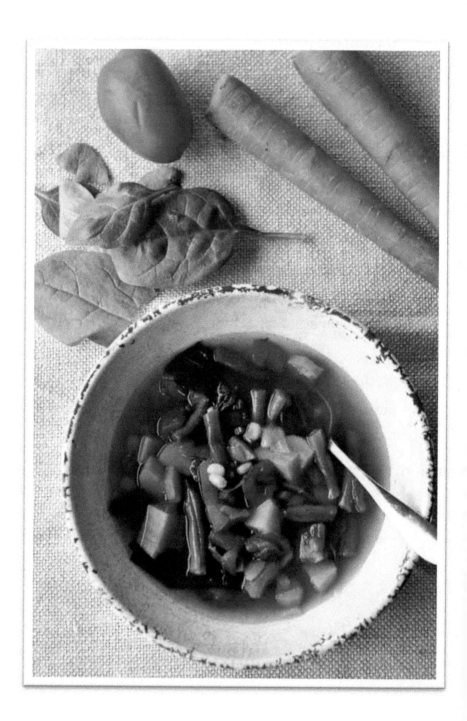

The Mediterranean Delight with Fresh Vinaigrette

Preparation Time: 5 minutes

Cooking Time: 10 minutes

Servings: 2

Ingredients:

- Herbed citrus vinaigrette:
- 1 tablespoon of lemon juice
- 2 tablespoons of orange juice
- ½ teaspoon of lemon zest
- ½ teaspoon of orange zest
- 2 tablespoons of olive oil
- 1 tablespoon of finely chopped fresh oregano leaves
- Salt to taste
- Black pepper to taste
- 2-3 tablespoons of freshly julienned mint leaves
- Salad:
- 1 freshly diced medium-sized cucumber

- 2 cups of cooked and rinsed chickpeas

- ½ cup of freshly diced red onion

- 2 freshly diced medium-sized tomatoes

- 1 freshly diced red bell pepper

- ¼ cup of green olives

- ½ cup of pomegranates

Directions:

1. In a large salad bowl, add the juice and zest of both the lemon and the orange along with oregano and olive oil. Whisk together so that they are mixed well. Season the vinaigrette with salt and pepper to taste.

2. After draining the chickpeas, add them to the dressing. Then, add the onions. Give them a thorough mix, so that the onion and chickpeas absorb the flavors.

3. Now, chop the rest of the veggies and start adding them to the salad bowl. Give them a good toss.

4. Lastly, add the olives and fresh mint. Adjust the salt and pepper as required.

5. Serve this Mediterranean delight chilled — a cool summer salad that is good for the tummy and the soul.

Nutrition: Kcal: 286 Carbohydrates: 29 g Protein: 1 g Fat: 11 g

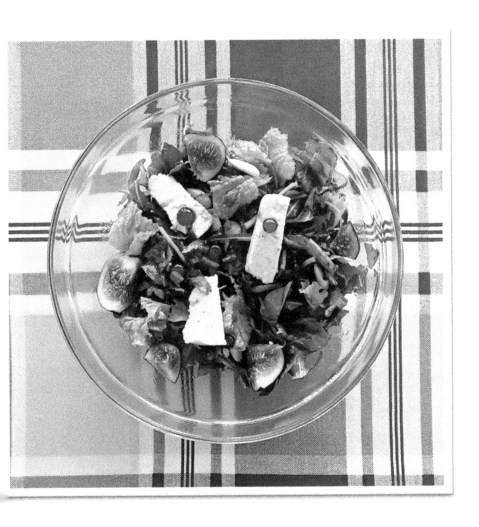

Chickpea and Mayonnaise Salad Sandwich

Preparation Time: 10 minutes

Cooking Time: 0 minutes

Servings: 4

Ingredients:

For the mayonnaise:

- 1/3 cup cashew nuts, soaked in boiling water for 10 minutes
- ½ teaspoon ground black pepper
- 1 teaspoon salt
- 6 teaspoons apple cider vinegar
- 2 teaspoon maple syrup
- 1/2 teaspoon Dijon mustard

For the chickpea salad:

- 1 small bunch of chives, chopped
- 1 ½ cup sweetcorn
- 3 cups cooked chickpeas

To serve:

- 4 sandwich bread

- 4 leaves of lettuce

- ½ cup chopped cherry tomatoes

Directions:

1. Prepare the mayonnaise and for this, place all of its ingredients in a food processor and then pulse for 2 minutes until smooth, scraping the sides of the container frequently.

2. Take a medium bowl, place chickpeas in it, and then mash by using a fork until broken.

3. Add chives and corn, stir until mixed, then add mayonnaise and stir until well combined.

4. Assemble the sandwich and for this, stuff sandwich bread with chickpea salad, top each sandwich with a lettuce leaf, and ¼ cup of chopped tomatoes and then serve.

Nutrition: 387 Cal 19 g Fat 5 g Saturated Fat 39.7 g Carbohydrates 7.2 g Fiber 4.6 g Sugars 10 g Protein

Cheesy Macaroni with Broccoli

Preparation Time: 10 minutes

Cooking Time: 25 minutes

Servings: 6

Ingredients

- 1/3 cup melted coconut oil

- ¼ cup nutritional yeast

- 1 tablespoon tomato paste

- 1 tablespoon dried mustard

- 2 garlic cloves, minced

- 1 ½ teaspoons salt

- ½ teaspoon ground turmeric

- 4 ½ cups almond milk

- 3 cups cauliflower florets, chopped

- 1 cup raw cashews, chopped

- 1 lb. shell pasta

- 1 tablespoon white vinegar

- 3 cups broccoli florets

Directions:

1. Place a suitably-sized saucepan over medium heat and add coconut oil.

2. Stir in mustard, yeast, garlic, salt, tomato paste, and turmeric.

3. Cook for 1 minute then add almond milk, cashews, and cauliflower florets.

4. Continue cooking for 20 minutes on a simmer.

5. Transfer the cauliflower mixture to a blender jug then blend until smooth.

6. Stir in vinegar and blend until creamy.

7. Fill a suitably-sized pot with salted water and bring it to a boil on high heat.

8. Add pasta to the boiling water.

9. Place a steamer basket over the boiling water and add broccoli to the basket.

10. Cook until the pasta is al dente. Drain and rinse the pasta and transfer the broccoli to a bowl.

11. Add the cooked pasta to the cauliflower-cashews sauce.

12. Toss in broccoli florets, salt, and black pepper.

13. Mix well then serve.

Nutrition: Calories: 40; Fat: 2.0g Protein: 5g Carbohydrates: 7g Fiber: 4g Sugar: 3g Sodium: 18mg

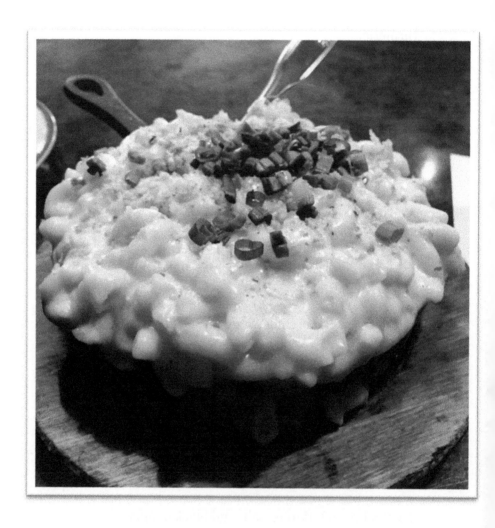

Crunchy Peanut Butter Apple Dip

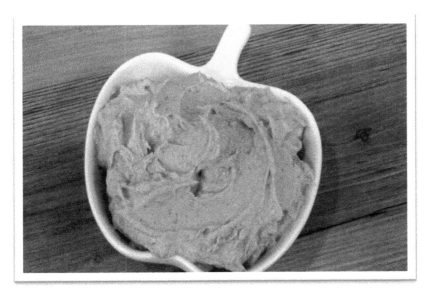

Preparation Time: 10 minutes

Cooking Time: 10 minutes

Servings: 2

Ingredients:

- 1 carton (8 oz.) reduced-fat spreadable cream cheese

- 1 cup creamy peanut butter

- 1/4 cup coconut milk

- 1 tablespoon brown sugar

- 1 teaspoon vanilla extract

- 1/2 cup chopped unsalted peanuts

- Apple slices

Directions:

1. Beat the initial 5 ingredients in a small bowl until combined. Mix in peanuts. Serve with slices of apple, then put the leftovers in the fridge.

Nutrition: Calories 125 Fat 5 Carbs 23 Protein 9

Creamy Cucumber Yogurt Dip

Preparation Time: 15 minutes

Cooking Time: 15 minutes

Servings: 4

Ingredients:

- 1 cup (8 oz.) reduced-fat plain yogurt

- 4 oz. reduced-fat cream cheese

- 1/2 cup chopped seeded peeled cucumber

- 1-1/2 teaspoon. finely chopped onion

- 1-1/2 teaspoon. snipped fresh dill or 1/2 teaspoon dill weed

- 1 teaspoon lemon juice

- 1 teaspoon grated lemon peel

- 1 garlic clove, minced

- 1/4 teaspoon salt

- 1/4 teaspoon pepper

- Assorted fresh vegetables

Directions:

1. Mix the cream cheese and yogurt in a small bowl. Stir in pepper, salt, garlic, peel, lemon juice, dill, onion, and cucumber. Put on the cover and let it chill in the fridge. Serve it with the veggies.

Nutrition: Calories 55 Fat 4 Carbs 12 Protein 6

Creamy Vegan Mushroom Pasta

Preparation Time: 10 minutes

Cooking Time: 30 minutes

Servings: 6

Ingredients:

- 2 cups frozen peas, thawed
- 3 tablespoons flour, unbleached
- 3 cups almond breeze, unsweetened
- 1 tablespoon nutritional yeast
- 1/3 cup fresh parsley, chopped, plus extra for garnish
- ¼ cup olive oil
- 1 pound pasta of choice
- 4 cloves garlic, minced
- 2/3 cup shallots, chopped
- 8 cups mixed mushrooms, sliced
- Salt and black pepper, to taste

Directions:

1. Take a bowl and boil pasta in salted water.

2. Heat olive oil in a pan over medium heat.

3. Add mushrooms, garlic, shallots and ½ tsp salt and cook for 15 minutes.

4. Sprinkle flour on the vegetables and stir for a minute while cooking.

5. Add almond beverage, stir constantly.

6. Let it simmer for 5 minutes and add pepper to it.

7. Cook for 3 more minutes and remove from heat.

8. Stir in nutritional yeast.

9. Add peas, salt, and pepper.

10. Cook for another minute and add

11. Add pasta to this sauce.

12. Garnish and serve!

Nutrition: Calories: 364 Total Fat: 28g Protein: 24g Total Carbs: 4g Fiber: 2g Net Carbs: 2g

Paprika Sweet Potato

Preparation Time: 10 minutes

Cooking Time: 11 minutes

Servings: 2

Ingredients:

- 2 sweet potatoes
- 2 teaspoons sweet paprika
- 1/2 teaspoon oregano, dried
- 1 teaspoon chili powder
- 1 teaspoon chives, chopped
- 1/2 cup of water

Directions:

1. Pour water in the instant pot and insert steamer rack.
2. Put potatoes on the rack and close the lid.
3. Set Manual mode (High pressure) and cook for 11 minutes. Then use quick pressure release.
4. Transfer the potatoes on the plate, cut into halves, sprinkle the rest of the Ingredients on top and serve.

Nutrition: Calories: 159, Fat: 3.4, Fiber: 2.8, Carbs: 33.8, Protein: 3.6

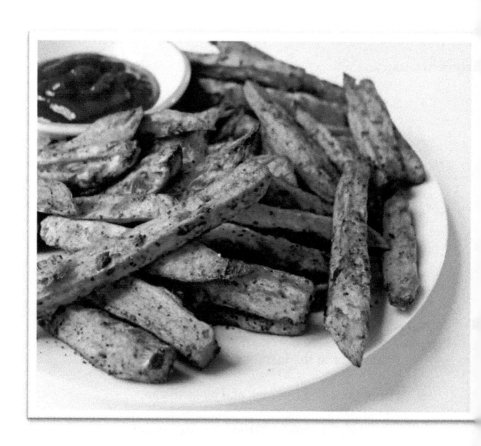

Wild Rice and Corn

Preparation Time: 10 minutes

Cooking Time: 8 minutes

Servings: 4

Ingredients:

- 1 cup wild rice
- 1 tablespoon Italian seasoning
- 1/4 cup corn kernels, canned
- 1 teaspoon chili powder
- 1 teaspoon salt
- 2 cups vegetable broth
- 1 tablespoon chives, chopped
- 2 tablespoons olive oil

Directions:

1. Pour olive oil in the instant pot and set Saute mode.
2. Add rice and seasoning and cook for 2 minutes.
3. Add the rest of the Ingredients and toss.
4. Set Manual mode (High pressure) and close the lid. Seal it.

5. Cook rice for 6 minutes. Use quick pressure release.

Nutrition: Calories: 254 Fat: 4.3 Fiber: 1.5 Carbs: 25.4 Protein: 5.4

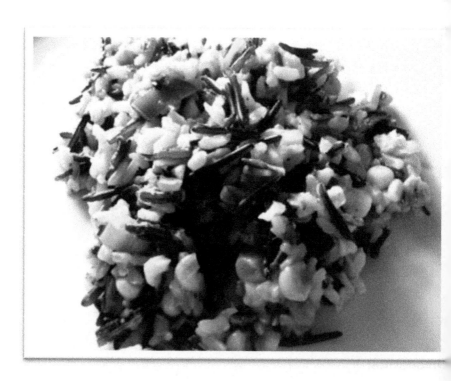

Kale Polenta

Preparation Time: 5 minutes

Cooking Time: 8 minutes

Servings: 5

Ingredients:

- 1 cup polenta

- 1/2 cup kale, chopped

- 1 teaspoon turmeric powder

- 1 teaspoon smoked paprika

- 4 cups vegetable broth

- 2 tablespoons coconut milk

- 1/2 teaspoon ground black pepper

- 1 teaspoon salt

Directions:

1. Whisk together polenta and vegetable broth.

2. Pour mixture in the instant pot, add the rest of the Ingredients and toss.

3. Close the lid and cook it on Manual mode (High pressure) for 8 minutes. Use quick pressure release/

4. Transfer cooked polenta in the bowl, stir and serve.

Nutrition: Calories: 182, Fat: 2.8, Fiber: 1, Carbs: 20.5, Protein: 6.3

Tomato Gazpacho

Preparation Time: 30 minutes

Cooking Time: 55 minutes

Servings: 6

Ingredients:

- 2 Tablespoons + 1 Teaspoon Red Wine Vinegar, Divided

- ½ Teaspoon Pepper

- 1 Teaspoon Sea Salt

- 1 Avocado,

- ¼ Cup Basil, Fresh & Chopped

- 3 Tablespoons + 2 Teaspoons Olive Oil, Divided

- 1 Clove Garlic, crushed

- 1 Red Bell Pepper, Sliced & Seeded

- 1 Cucumber, Chunked

- 2 ½ lbs. Large Tomatoes, Cored & Chopped

Directions:

1. Place half of your cucumber, bell pepper, and ¼ cup of each tomato in a bowl, covering. Set it in the fried.

2. Puree your remaining tomatoes, cucumber and bel
   pepper with garlic, three tablespoons oil, two tablespoon:
   of vinegar, sea salt and black pepper into a blender
   blending until smooth. Transfer it to a bowl, and chill fo:
   two hours.

3. Chop the avocado, adding it to your chopped vegetables
   adding your remaining oil, vinegar, salt, pepper and basil.

4. Ladle your tomato puree mixture into bowls, and serve
   with chopped vegetables as a salad.

5. Interesting Facts:

6. Avocados themselves are ranked within the top five of the
   healthiest foods on the planet, so you know that the oi:
   that is produced from them is too. It is loaded with healthy
   fats and essential fatty acids. Like race bran oil it is perfec
   to cook with as well! Bonus: Helps in the prevention o:
   diabetes and lowers cholesterol levels.

Nutrition: Calories 201 Protein 23g Fat 4 Carbs 2

Tomato Pumpkin Soup

Preparation Time: 25 minutes

Cooking Time: 25 minutes

Servings: 4

Ingredients:

- 2 cups pumpkin, diced

- 1/2 cup tomato, chopped

- 1/2 cup onion, chopped

- 1 1/2 tsp curry powder

- 1/2 tsp paprika

- 2 cups vegetable stock

- 1 tsp olive oil

- 1/2 tsp garlic, minced

Directions:

1. In a saucepan, add oil, garlic, and onion and sauté for 3 minutes over medium heat.

2. Add remaining ingredients into the saucepan and bring to boil.

3. Reduce heat and cover and simmer for 10 minutes.

4. Puree the soup using a blender until smooth.

5. Stir well and serve warm.

Nutrition: Calories: 340 Protein: 50 g Carbohydrate: 14 g Fat: 10g

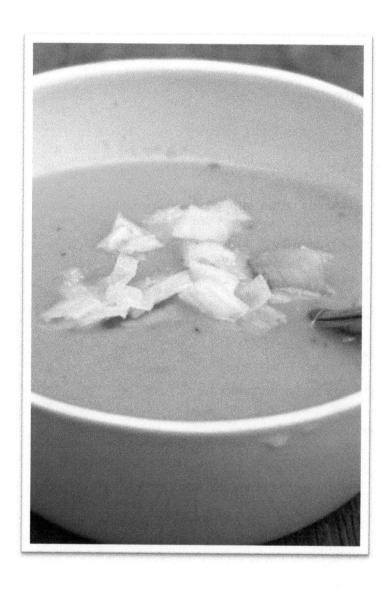

Creamy Garlic Onion Soup

Preparation Time: 45 minutes

Cooking Time: 25 minutes

Servings: 4

Ingredients:

- 1 onion, sliced

- 4 cups vegetable stock

- 1 1/2 tbsp. olive oil

- 1 shallot, sliced

- 2 garlic clove, chopped

- 1 leek, sliced

- Salt

Directions:

1. Add stock and olive oil in a saucepan and bring to boil.

2. Add remaining ingredients and stir well.

3. Cover and simmer for 25 minutes.

4. Puree the soup using an immersion blender until smooth.

5. Stir well and serve warm.

Nutrition: Calories 115 Protein 30g Fat 0 Carbs 3

Chocolate and Hazelnut Smoothie

Preparation Time: 5 minutes

Cooking Time: 0 minutes

Servings: 4

Ingredients:

- 1 frozen banana

- 1 cup hazelnuts, unsalted, roasted

- 8 teaspoons maple syrup

- 4 tablespoons cocoa powder, unsweetened

- 1/2 teaspoon hazelnut extract, unsweetened

- 2 cups almond milk, unsweetened

- 1 cup of ice cubes

Directions:

1. Add all the ingredients in the order into a food processor or blender and then pulse for 1 to 2 minutes until blended, scraping the sides of the container frequently.

2. Distribute the smoothie among glasses and then serve.

Nutrition: 198 Cal 12 g Fat 1 g Saturated Fat 21 g Carbohydrates 5 g Fiber 12 g Sugars 5 g Protein

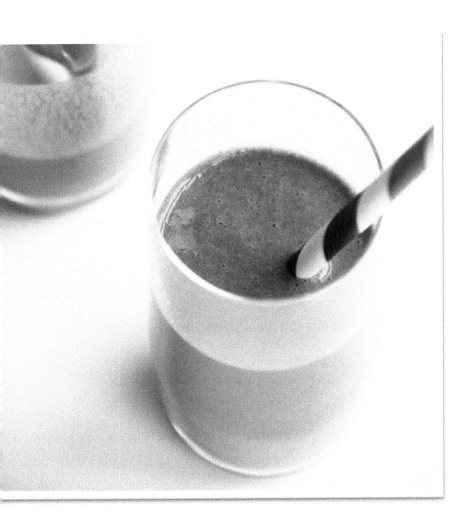

Blueberry Oatmeal Smoothie

Preparation Time: 5 minutes

Cooking Time: 0 minutes

Servings: 4

Ingredients:

- 2 cups frozen blueberries

- 1 cup old-fashioned oats

- 2 teaspoons cinnamon

- 2 tablespoons maple syrup

- 1 cup spinach

- 2 cup almond milk, unsweetened

- 8 ice cubes

Directions:

1. Add all the ingredients in the order into a food processor or blender and then pulse for 1 to 2 minutes until blended scraping the sides of the container frequently.

2. Distribute the smoothie among glasses and then serve.

Nutrition: 194 Cal 5 g Fat 3 g Saturated Fat 34 g Carbohydrates 5 g Fiber 15 g Sugars 5 g Protein

Orange French Toast

Preparation Time: 5 minutes

Cooking Time: 30 minutes

Servings: 8 servings

Ingredients:

- 2 cups of plant milk (unflavored)
- Four tablespoon maple syrup
- 11/2 tablespoon cinnamon
- Salt (optional)
- 1 cup flour (almond)
- 1 tablespoon orange zest
- 8 bread slices

Directions:

1. Turn the oven and heat to 400 degree F afterwards.
2. In a cup, add **Ingredients:** and whisk until the batter is smooth.
3. Dip each piece of bread into the paste and permit to soak for a couple of seconds.
4. Put in the pan, and cook until lightly browned.

5. Put the toast on the cookie sheet and bake for ten to fifteen minutes in the oven, until it is crispy.

Nutrition: Calories: 129 Fat: 1.1g Carbohydrates: 21.5g Protein: 7.9g

Veggie Noodles

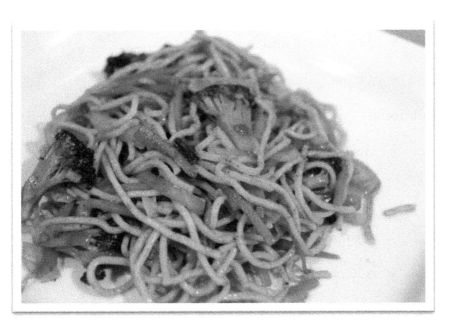

Preparation Time: 10 minutes

Cooking Time: 5 minutes

Servings: 2

Ingredients:

- 2 tablespoons vegetable oil

- 4 spring onions, divided

- 1 cup snap pea

- 2 tablespoons brown sugar

- 9 oz. dried rice noodles, cooked

- 5 garlic cloves, minced

- 2 carrots, cut into small sticks

- 3 tablespoons soy sauce

Directions:

1. Heat vegetable oil in a skillet over medium heat and add garlic and 3 spring onions.

2. Cook for about 3 minutes and add the carrots, peas, brown sugar and soy sauce.

3. Add rice noodles and cook for about 2 minutes.

4. Season with salt and black pepper and top with remaining spring onion to serve.

Nutrition: Calories: 25; Fat: 2.0g Protein: 5.2g Carbohydrates: 5.3g Fiber: 4g; Sodium: 18mg

Minutes Vegetarian Pasta

Preparation Time: 5 minutes

Cooking Time: 16 minutes

Servings: 4

Ingredients:

- 3 shallots, chopped

- ¼ teaspoon red pepper flakes

- ¼ cup vegan parmesan cheese

- 2 tablespoons olive oil

- 2 garlic cloves, minced

- 8-ounces spinach leaves

- 8-ounces linguine pasta

- 1 pinch salt

- 1 pinch black pepper

Directions:

1. Boil salted water in a large pot and add pasta.

2. Cook for about 6 minutes and drain the pasta in a colander.

3. Heat olive oil over medium heat in a large skillet and add the shallots.

4. Cook for about 5 minutes until soft and caramelized and stir in the spinach, garlic, red pepper flakes, salt and black pepper.

5. Cook for about 5 minutes and add pasta and 2 ladles of pasta water.

6. Stir in the parmesan cheese and dish out in a bowl to serve.

Nutrition: Calories: 25; Fat: 2.0g Protein: 5.2g Carbohydrates: 5.3g Fiber: 4g; Sodium: 18mg

Pesto Quinoa with White Beans

Preparation Time: 5 minutes

Cooking Time: 15 minutes

Servings: 4

Ingredients:

- 12 ounces cooked white bean

- 3 ½ cups quinoa, cooked

- 1 medium zucchini, sliced

- ¾ cup sun-dried tomato

- ¼ cup pine nuts

- 1 tablespoon olive oil

For the Pesto:

- 1/3 cup walnuts

- 2 cups arugula

- 1 teaspoon minced garlic

- 2 cups basil

- ¾ teaspoon salt

- ¼ teaspoon ground black pepper

- 1 tablespoon lemon juice

- 1/3 cup olive oil

- 2 tablespoons water

Directions:

1. Prepare the pesto, and for this, place all of its ingredient in a food processor and pulse for 2 minutes until smooth scraping the sides of the container frequently and set asid until required.

2. Take a large skillet pan, place it over medium heat, add oi and when hot, add zucchini and cook for 4 minutes unti tender-crisp.

3. Season zucchini with salt and black pepper, cook for minutes until lightly brown, then add tomatoes and whit beans and continue cooking for 4 minutes until whit beans begin to crisp.

4. Stir in pine nuts, cook for 2 minutes until toasted, the remove the pan from heat and transfer zucchini mixtur into a medium bowl.

5. Add quinoa and pesto, stir until well combined, the distribute among four bowls and then serve.

Nutrition: 352 Cal 27.3 g Fat 5 g Saturated Fat 33.7 g Carbohydrate 5.7 g Fiber 4.5 g Sugars 9.7 g Protein

Spicy Carrots and Olives

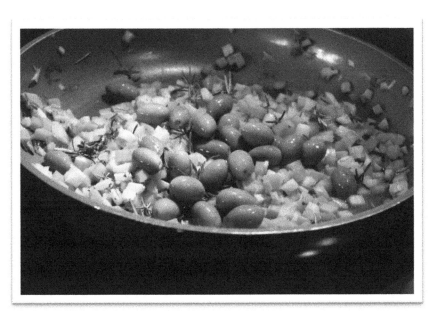

Preparation Time: 15 minutes

Cooking Time: 10 minutes

Servings: 4

Ingredients:

- ½ teaspoon hot paprika

- 1 red chili pepper, minced

- ¼ teaspoon ground cumin

- ¼ teaspoon dried oregano

- ¼ teaspoon dried basil

- ½ teaspoon salt

- 1 tablespoon olive oil

- 1 pound baby carrots, peeled

- 1 cup kalamata olives, pitted and halved

- juice of 1 lime

Directions:

1. Heat up a pan with the oil over medium heat, add the carrots, olives and the other ingredients, toss, cook for 10 minutes, divide between plates and serve.

Nutrition: Calories 141 Fat 5.8 Fiber 4.3 Carbs 7.5 Protein 9.6

Tamarind Avocado Bowls

Preparation Time: 10 minutes

Cooking Time: 0 minutes

Servings: 2

Ingredients:

- 1 teaspoon cumin seeds

- 1 tablespoon olive oil

- ½ teaspoon gram masala

- 1 teaspoon ground ginger

- 2 avocados, peeled, pitted and roughly cubed

- 1 mango, peeled, and cubed

- 1 cup cherry tomatoes, halved

- ½ teaspoon cayenne pepper

- 1 teaspoon turmeric powder

- 3 tablespoons tamarind paste

Directions:

1. In a bowl, mix the avocados with the mango and the other ingredients, toss and serve.

Nutrition: Calories 170 Fat 4.5 Fiber 3 Carbs 5 Protein 6

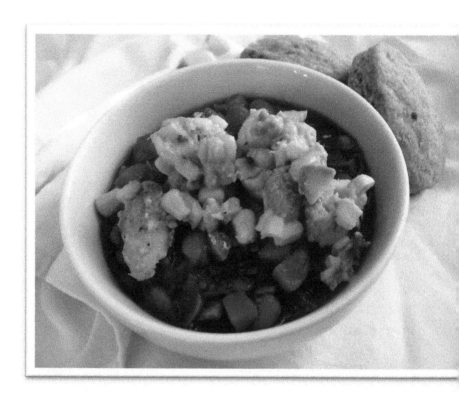

Avocado and Leeks Mix

Preparation Time: 10 minutes

Cooking Time: 0 minutes

Servings: 4

Ingredients:

- 1 small red onion, chopped

- 2 avocados, pitted, peeled and chopped

- 1 teaspoon chili powder

- 2 leeks, sliced

- 1 cup cucumber, cubed

- 1 cup cherry tomatoes, halved

- Salt and black pepper to the taste

- 2 tablespoons cumin powder

- 2 tablespoons lime juice

- 1 tablespoon parsley, chopped

Directions:

1. In a bowl, mix the onion with the avocados, chili powder and the other ingredients, toss and serve.

Nutrition: Calories 120 Fat 2 Fiber 2 Carbs 7 Protein 4

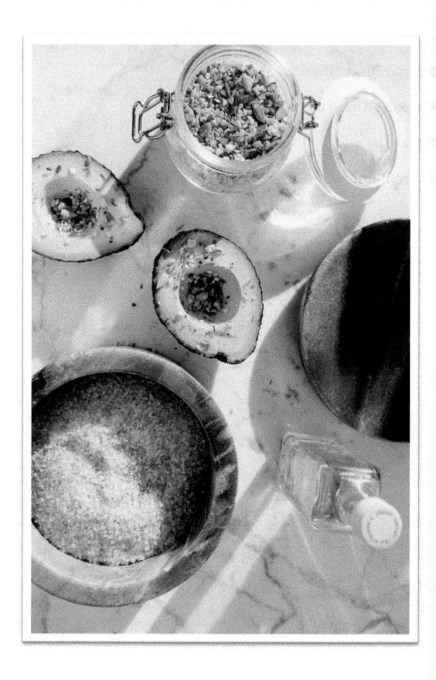

Cabbage Bowls

Preparation Time: 10 minutes

Cooking Time: 10 minutes

Servings: 4

Ingredients:

- 1 green cabbage head, shredded

- 1 red cabbage head, shredded

- 1 teaspoon garam masala

- 1 teaspoon basil, dried

- 1 teaspoon coriander, ground

- 1 teaspoon mustard seeds

- 1 tablespoon balsamic vinegar

- ¼ cup tomatoes, crushed

- A pinch of salt and black pepper

- 3 carrots, shredded

- 1 yellow bell pepper, chopped

- 1 orange bell pepper, chopped

- 1 red bell pepper, chopped

- 2 tablespoons dill, chopped

- 2 tablespoons olive oil

Directions:

1. Heat up a pan with the oil over medium heat, add the peppers and carrots and cook for 2 minutes.

2. Add the cabbage and the other ingredients, toss, cook for 10 minutes, divide between plates and serve.

Nutrition: Calories 150 Fat 9 Fiber 4 Carbs 3.3 Protein 4.4

Pomegranate and Pears Salad

Preparation Time: 10 minutes

Cooking Time: 0 minutes

Servings: 3

Ingredients:

- 3 big pears, cored and cut with a spiralizer

- ¾ cup pomegranate seeds

- 2 cups baby spinach

- ½ cup black olives, pitted and cubed

- ¾ cup walnuts, chopped1 tablespoon olive oil

- 1 tablespoon coconut sugar

- 1 teaspoon white sesame seeds

- 2 tablespoons chives, chopped

- 1 tablespoon balsamic vinegar

- 1 garlic clove, minced

- A pinch of sea salt and black pepper

Directions:

1. In a bowl, mix the pears with the pomegranate seeds, spinach and the other ingredients, toss and serve.

Nutrition: Calories 200 Fat 3.9 Fiber 4 Carbs 6 Protein 3.3

Bulgur and Tomato Mix

Preparation Time: 15 minutes

Cooking Time: 0 minutes

Servings: 4

Ingredients:

- 1 ½ cups hot water

- 1 cup bulgur

- Juice of 1 lime

- 1 cup cherry tomatoes, halved

- 4 tablespoons cilantro, chopped

- ½ cup cranberries, dried

- juice of ½ lemon

- 1 teaspoon oregano, dried

- 1/3 cup almonds, sliced

- ¼ cup green onions, chopped

- ½ cup red bell peppers, chopped

- ½ cup carrots, grated

- 1 tablespoon avocado oil

- A pinch of sea salt and black pepper

Directions:

1. Place bulgur into a bowl, add boiling water to it, stir, and cover and set aside for 15 minutes.

2. Fluff bulgur with a fork and transfer to a bowl.

3. Add the rest of the ingredients, toss and serve.

Nutrition: Calories 260 Fat 4.4 Fiber 3 Carbs 7 Protein 10

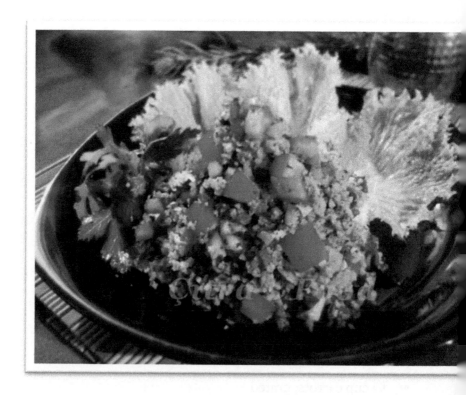

Mushroom Steaks

Preparation Time: 10 minutes

Cooking Time: 24 minutes

Servings: 4

Ingredients:

- 1 tablespoon vegan butter

- ½ cup vegetable broth

- ½ small yellow onion, diced

- 1 large garlic clove, minced

- 3 tablespoons balsamic vinegar

- 1 tablespoon mirin

- ½ tablespoon soy sauce

- ½ tablespoon tomato paste

- 1 teaspoon dried thyme

- ½ teaspoon dried basil

- A dash of ground black pepper

- 2 large, whole portobello mushrooms

Directions:

1. Melt butter in a saucepan over medium heat and stir in half of the broth.

2. Bring to a simmer then add garlic and onion. Cook for 8 minutes.

3. Whisk the rest of the ingredients except the mushrooms in a bowl.

4. Add this mixture to the onion in the pan and mix well.

5. Bring this filling to a simmer then remove from the heat.

6. Clean the mushroom caps inside and out and divide the filling between the mushrooms.

7. Place the mushrooms on a baking sheet and top them with remaining sauce and broth.

8. Cover with foil then place it on a grill to smoke.

9. Cover the grill and broil for 16 minutes over indirect heat.

10. Serve warm.

Nutrition: Calories: 887 Total Fat: 93g Carbs: 29g Net Carbs: 13g Fiber: 4g Protein: 8g

Chunky Cucumber Salsa

Preparation Time: 20 minutes

Cooking Time: 20 minutes

Servings: 4

Ingredients:

- 3 medium cucumbers, peeled and coarsely chopped
- 1 medium mango, coarsely chopped
- 1 cup frozen corn, thawed
- 1 medium sweet red pepper, coarsely chopped
- 1 small red onion, coarsely chopped
- 1 jalapeno pepper, finely chopped
- 3 garlic cloves, minced
- 2 tablespoon white wine vinegar
- 1 tablespoon minced fresh cilantro
- 1 teaspoon salt
- 1/2 teaspoon sugar
- 1/4 to 1/2 teaspoon cayenne pepper

Directions:

1. Mix all ingredients in a big bowl, then chill, covered, about 2 to 3 hours before serving.

Nutrition: Calories 215 Fat 5 Carbs 23 Protein 10

Low-fat Stuffed Mushrooms

Preparation Time: 20 minutes

Cooking Time: 25 minutes

Servings: 6

Ingredients:

- 1 lb. large fresh mushrooms

- 3 tablespoons seasoned bread crumbs

- 3 tablespoons fat-free sour cream

- 2 tablespoons grated Parmesan cheese

- 2 tablespoons minced chives

- 2 tablespoons reduced-fat mayonnaise

- 2 teaspoons balsamic vinegar

- 2 to 3 drops hot pepper sauce, optional

Directions:

1. Take out the stems from the mushrooms, then put the cups aside. Chop the stems and set aside 1/3 cup (get rid of the leftover stems or reserve for later use).

2. Mix the reserved mushroom stems, hot pepper sauce if preferred, vinegar, mayonnaise, chives, Parmesan cheese, sour cream, and breadcrumbs in a bowl, then stir well.

3. Put the mushroom caps on a cooking spray-coated baking tray and stuff it with the crumb mixture.

4. Let it boil for 5 to 7 minutes, placed 4-6 inches from the heat source, or until it turns light brown.

Nutrition: Calories 435 Fat 4 Carbs 23 Protein 9

Vegetable Penne Pasta

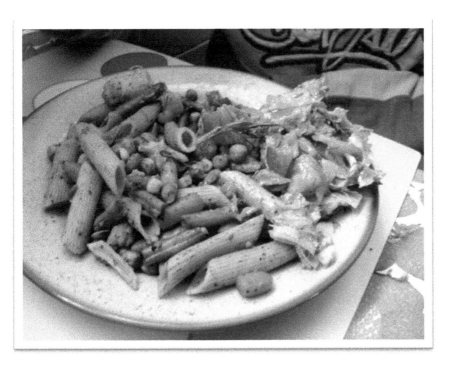

Preparation Time: 15 minutes

Cooking Time: 20 minutes

Servings: 6

Ingredients:

- ½ large onion, chopped

- 2 celery sticks, chopped

82

- ½ tablespoon ginger paste

- ½ cup green bell pepper

- 1½ tablespoons soy sauce

- ½ teaspoon parsley

- Salt and black pepper, to taste

- ½ pound penne pasta, cooked

- 2 large carrots, diced

- ½ small leek, chopped

- 1 tablespoon olive oil

- ½ teaspoon garlic paste

- ½ tablespoon Worcester sauce

- ½ teaspoon coriander

- 1 cup water

Directions:

1. Heat olive oil in a wok on medium heat and add onions, garlic and ginger paste.

2. Sauté for about 3 minutes and stir in all bell pepper, celery sticks, carrots and leek.

3. Sauté for about 5 minutes and add remaining ingredients except for pasta.

4. Cover the lid and cook for about 12 minutes.

5. Stir in the cooked pasta and dish out to serve warm.

Nutrition: Calories: 385 Total Fat: 29g Protein: 26g Total Carbs: 5g Fiber: 1g Net Carbs: 4g

Minted Peas

Preparation Time: 5 minutes

Cooking Time: 5 minutes

Servings: 4

Ingredients:

- 1 tablespoon olive oil

- 4 cups peas, fresh or frozen (not canned)

- ½ teaspoon sea salt

- freshly ground black pepper

- 3 tablespoons chopped fresh mint

Directions:

1. In a large sauté pan, heat the olive oil over medium-high heat until hot. Add the peas and cook, about 5 minutes.

2. Remove the pan from heat. Stir in the salt, season with pepper, and stir in the mint.

3. Serve hot.

Nutrition: Calories: 77Fat: 3gProtein: 4gCarbohydrates: 12gFiber: 5gSugar: 3gSodium: 320mg

Glazed Curried Carrots

Preparation Time: 5 minutes

Cooking Time: 15 minutes

Servings: 6

Ingredients:

- 1-pound carrots, peeled and thinly sliced

- 2 tablespoons olive oil

- 2 tablespoons curry powder

- 2 tablespoons pure maple syrup

- juice of ½ lemon

- sea salt

- freshly ground black pepper

Directions:

1. Place the carrots in a large pot and cover with water. Cook on medium-high heat until tender, about 10 minutes. Drain the carrots and return them to the pan over medium-low heat.

2. Stir in the olive oil, curry powder, maple syrup, and lemon juice. Cook, stirring constantly, until the liquid reduces,

about 5 minutes. Season with salt and pepper and serve immediately.

Nutrition: Calories: 171Fat: 3gProtein: 4gCarbohydrates: 34gFiber: 5gSugar: 3gSodium: 129mg

Thai Roasted Broccoli

Preparation Time: 5 minutes

Cooking Time: 15 minutes

Servings: 4

Ingredients:

- 1 head broccoli, cut into florets

- 2 tablespoons olive oil

- 1 tablespoon soy sauce or gluten-free tamari

Directions:

1. Preheat the oven to 425°F. Line a baking sheet with parchment paper. In a large bowl, combine the broccoli, oil, and soy sauce. Toss well to combine.

2. Spread the broccoli on the prepared baking sheet. Roast for 10 minutes.

3. Toss the broccoli with a spatula and roast for an additional 5 minutes, or until the edges of the florets begin to brown.

Nutrition: Calories: 44Fat: 2gProtein: 3gCarbohydrates: 7gFiber: 2gSugar: 3gSodium: 20mg

Coconut Curry Noodle

Preparation Time: 10 minutes

Cooking Time: 30 minutes

Servings: 4

Ingredients:

- ½ tablespoon oil

- 3 garlic cloves, minced

- 2 tablespoons lemongrass, minced

- 1 tablespoon fresh ginger, grated

- 2 tablespoons red curry paste

- 1 (14 oz.) can coconut milk

- 1 tablespoon brown sugar

- 2 tablespoons soy sauce

- 2 tablespoons fresh lime juice

- 1 tablespoon hot chili paste

- 12 oz. linguine

- 2 cups broccoli florets

- 1 cup carrots, shredded

- 1 cup edamame, shelled

- 1 red bell pepper, sliced

Directions:

1. Fill a suitably-sized pot with salted water and boil it on high heat.

2. Add pasta to the boiling water and cook until it is al dente then rinse under cold water.

3. Now place a medium-sized saucepan over medium heat and add oil.

4. Stir in ginger, garlic, and lemongrass, then sauté for 30 seconds.

5. Add coconut milk, soy sauce, curry paste, brown sugar, chili paste, and lime juice.

6. Stir this curry mixture for 10 minutes, or until it thickens.

7. Toss in carrots, broccoli, edamame, bell pepper, and cooked pasta.

8. Mix well, then serve warm.

Nutrition: Calories: 44Fat: 2gProtein: 3gCarbohydrates: 7gFiber: 2gSugar: 3gSodium: 20mg

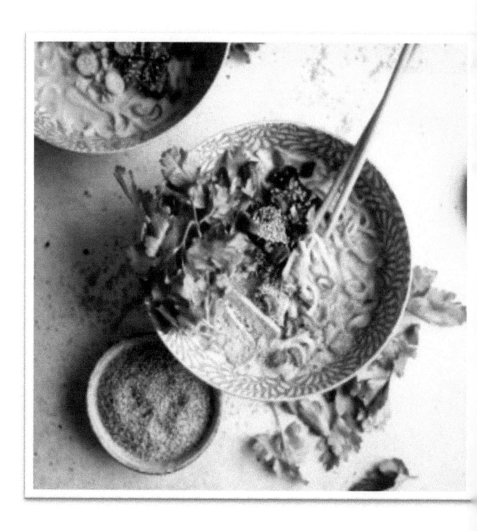

Collard Green Pasta

Preparation Time: 10 minutes

Cooking Time: 20 minutes

Servings: 4

Ingredients

- 2 tablespoons olive oil

- 4 garlic cloves, minced

- 8 oz. whole wheat pasta

- ½ cup panko bread crumbs

- 1 tablespoon nutritional yeast

- 1 teaspoon red pepper flakes

- 1 large bunch collard greens

- 1 large lemon, zest and juiced

Directions:

1. Fill a suitable pot with salted water and boil it on high heat.

2. Add pasta to the boiling water and cook until it is al dente, then rinse under cold water.

3. Reserve ½ cup of the cooking liquid from the pasta.

4. Place a non-stick pan over medium heat and add 1 tablespoon olive oil.

5. Stir in half of the garlic, then sauté for 30 seconds.

6. Add breadcrumbs and sauté for approximately 5 minutes.

7. Toss in red pepper flakes and nutritional yeast then mix well.

8. Transfer the breadcrumbs mixture to a plate and clean the pan.

9. Add the remaining tablespoon oil to the nonstick pan.

10. Stir in the garlic clove, salt, black pepper, and chard leaves.

11. Cook for 5 minutes until the leaves are wilted.

12. Add pasta along with the reserved pasta liquid.

13. Mix well, then add garlic crumbs, lemon juice, and zest.

14. Toss well, then serve warm.

Nutrition: Calories: 45Fat: 2.5gProtein: 4gCarbohydrates: 9gFiber: 4gSugar: 3gSodium: 20mg

Glazed Avocado

Preparation Time: 10 minutes

Cooking Time: 12 minutes

Servings: 4

Ingredients:

- 1 tablespoon stevia

- 1 teaspoon olive oil

- 1 teaspoon water

- 1 teaspoon lemon juice

- ½ teaspoon rosemary, dried

- ½ teaspoon ground black pepper

- 2 avocados, peeled, pitted and cut into large pieces

Directions:

1. Heat up a pan with the oil over medium heat, add the avocados, stevia and the other ingredients, toss, cook for 12 minutes, divide into bowls and serve.

Nutrition: Calories 262 Fat 9.6 Fiber 0.1 Carbs 6.5 Protein 7.9

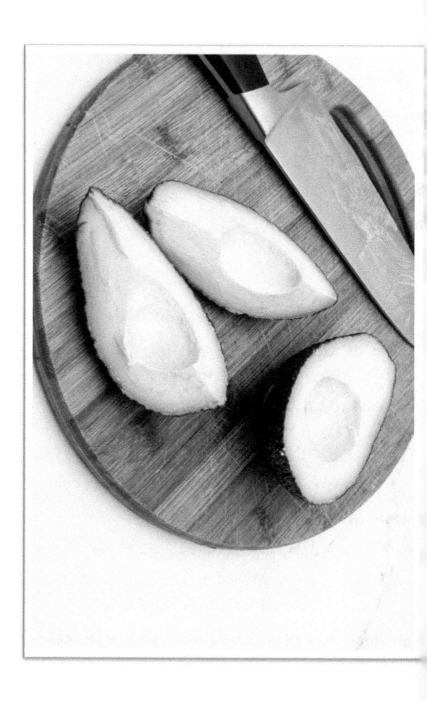

Mango and Leeks Meatballs

Preparation Time: 20 minutes

Cooking Time: 10 minutes

Servings: 4

Ingredients:

- 1 tablespoon mango puree
- 1 cup leeks, chopped
- ½ cup tofu, crumbled
- 1 teaspoon dried oregano
- 1 tablespoon almond flour
- 1 teaspoon olive oil
- 1 tablespoon flax meal
- ½ teaspoon chili flakes

Directions:

1. In the mixing bowl, mix up mango puree with leeks, tofu and the other ingredients except the oil and stir well.

2. Make the small meatballs.

3. After this, pour the olive oil in the skillet and heat it up.

4. Add the meatballs in the skillet and cook them for 4 minutes from each side.

Nutrition: Calories 147 Fat 8.6 Fiber 4.5 Carbs 5.6 Protein 5.3

Grilled Avocado Guacamole

Preparation Time: 10 minutes

Cooking Time: 20 minutes

Servings: 4

Ingredients:

- ½ teaspoon olive oil
- 1 lime, halved
- ½ onion, halved
- 1 serrano chile, halved, stemmed, and seeded
- 3 Haas avocados, skin on
- 2–3 tablespoons fresh cilantro, chopped
- ½ teaspoon smoked salt

Directions:

1. Preheat the grill over medium heat.
2. Brush the grilling grates with olive oil and place chile, onion, and lime on it.
3. Grill the onion for 10 minutes, chile for 5 minutes, and lime for 2 minutes.
4. Transfer the veggies to a large bowl.

5. Now cut the avocados in half and grill them for 5 minutes.

6. Mash the flesh of the grilled avocado in a bowl.

7. Chop the other grilled veggies and add them to the avocado mash.

8. Stir in remaining ingredients and mix well.

9. Serve.

Nutrition: Calories: 165 Total Fat: 17g Carbs: 4g Net Carbs: 2g Fiber: 1g Protein: 1g

Tofu Hoagie Rolls

Preparation Time: 10 minutes

Cooking Time: 20 minutes

Servings: 6

Ingredients:

- ½ cup vegetable broth

- ¼ cup hot sauce

- 1 tablespoon vegan butter

- 1 (16 ounce) package tofu, pressed and diced

- 4 cups cabbage, shredded

- 2 medium apples, grated

- 1 medium shallot, grated

- 6 tablespoons vegan mayonnaise

- 1 tablespoon apple cider vinegar

- Salt and black pepper

- 4 6-inch hoagie rolls, toasted

Directions:

1. In a saucepan, combine broth with butter and hot sauce and bring to a boil.

2. Add tofu and reduce the heat to a simmer.

3. Cook for 10 minutes then remove from heat and let sit for 10 minutes to marinate.

4. Toss cabbage and rest of the ingredients in a salad bowl.

5. Prepare and set up a grill on medium heat.

6. Drain the tofu and grill for 5 minutes per side.

7. Lay out the toasted hoagie rolls and add grilled tofu to each hoagie

8. Add the cabbage mixture evenly between them then close it.

9. Serve.

Nutrition: Calories: 111 Total Fat: 11g Carbs: 5g Net Carbs: 1g Fiber: 0g Protein: 1g

Beans Mix

Preparation Time: 10 minutes

Cooking Time: 15 minutes

Servings: 4

Ingredients:

- 1 ½ cups cooked black beans
- 1 cup cooked red kidney beans
- ½ teaspoon garlic powder
- ½ teaspoon smoked paprika
- 2 teaspoons chili powder
- 1 tablespoon olive oil
- 1 ½ cups chickpeas, cooked
- 1 teaspoon garam masala
- 1 red bell pepper, chopped
- 2 tomatoes, chopped
- 1 cup cashews, chopped
- ½ cup veggie stock
- 1 tablespoon balsamic vinegar

- 1 tablespoon oregano, chopped

- 1 tablespoon dill, chopped

- 1 cup corn kernels, chopped

Directions:

1. Heat up a pan with the oil over medium heat, add the beans, garlic powder, chili powder and the other ingredients, toss and cook for 15 minutes.

2. Divide between plates and serve.

Nutrition: Calories 300 Fat 8.3 Fiber 3.3 Carbs 6 Protein 13

Grilled Seitan with Creole Sauce

Preparation Time: 10 minutes

Cooking Time: 14 minutes

Servings: 4

Ingredients:

Grilled Seitan Kebabs:

- 4 cups seitan, diced

- 2 medium onions, diced into squares

- 8 bamboo skewers

- 1 can coconut milk

- 2½ tablespoons creole spice

- 2 tablespoons tomato paste

- 2 cloves of garlic

Creole Spice Mix:

- 2 tablespoons paprika

- 12 dried peri chili peppers

- 1 tablespoon salt

- 1 tablespoon freshly ground pepper

- 2 teaspoons dried thyme

- 2 teaspoons dried oregano

Directions:

1. Prepare the creole seasoning by blending all its ingredients and preserve in a sealable jar.

2. Thread seitan and onion on the bamboo skewers in an alternating pattern.

3. On a baking sheet, mix coconut milk with creole seasoning, tomato paste and garlic.

4. Soak the skewers in the milk marinade for 2 hours.

5. Prepare and set up a grill over medium heat.

6. Grill the skewers for 7 minutes per side.

7. Serve.

Nutrition: Calories: 407 Total Fat: 42g Carbs: 13g Net Carbs: 6g Fiber: 1g Protein: 4g